THE AFIB HEALING

COOKBOOK

GEORGE ANDERSON

The Author hereby reserves all rights provided by copyright law, including but not limited to the rights to reproduce, distribute, display, and create derivative works of the copyrighted book. Any unauthorized use, reproduction, or distribution of the book or its content without the express written consent of the Author is strictly prohibited and may result in legal action.

This Notice is without prejudice to any additional or more specific terms that may be included in a separate licensing agreement between the Author and a third party.

CHAPTER ONE

INTRODUCTION

What is AFib?

A diet rich in vegetables, whole grains, and legumes may help people reduce AFib episodes.

AFib is a type of arrhythmia that affects the upper chambers of the heart. The electrical impulses that control these chambers fire in a disorganized way, which leads to an irregular heartbeat.

AFib itself is not a life threatening condition. However, it can increase the risk of stroke, blood clots, and congestive heart failure.

Several possible risk factors increase the chances that someone will develop AFib. These include:

• having overweight

• diabetes

• high blood pressure (hypertension)

• smoking

• alcohol consumption

• obstructive sleep apnea

• high cholesterol

• having a family history of AFib

There is no cure for AFib. Some people may require medication, cardioversion, a pacemaker, or catheter ablation to manage the condition.

ARRHYTHMIA

Arrhythmias, also known as cardiac arrhythmias, heart arrhythmias, or dysrhythmias, are irregularities in the heartbeat, including when it is too fast or too slow. A heart rate that is too fast above 100 beats per minute in adults is called tachycardia, and a heart rate that is too slow below 60 beats per minute is called bradycardia. Some types of arrhythmias have no symptoms. Symptoms, when present, may include palpitations or feeling a pause between heartbeats. In more serious cases, there may be lightheadedness, passing out, shortness of breath or chest pain. While most cases of arrhythmia are not serious, some predispose a person to complications such as stroke or heart failure. Others may result in sudden death.

Arrhythmias are often categorized into four groups: extra beats, supraventricular tachycardias, ventricular arrhythmias and bradyarrhythmias. Extra beats include premature atrial contractions, premature ventricular contractions and premature junctional contractions. Supraventricular tachycardias include atrial fibrillation, atrial flutter and paroxysmal supraventricular tachycardia. Ventricular arrhythmias include ventricular fibrillation and ventricular tachycardia. Bradyarrhythmias are due to sinus node dysfunction or atrioventricular conduction disturbances. Arrhythmias are due to problems with the electrical conduction system of the heart. A number of tests can help with diagnosis, including an electrocardiogram (ECG) and Holter monitor.

Many arrhythmias can be effectively treated. Treatments may include medications, medical procedures such as inserting a pacemaker, and surgery. Medications for a fast heart rate may include beta blockers, or antiarrhythmic agents such as procainamide, which attempt to restore a normal heart rhythm. This latter group may have more significant side effects, especially if taken for a long period of time. Pacemakers are often used for slow heart rates. Those with an irregular heartbeat are often treated with blood thinners to reduce the risk of complications. Those who have severe symptoms from an arrhythmia or are medically unstable may receive urgent treatment with a controlled electric shock in the form of cardioversion or defibrillation.

Arrhythmia affects millions of people. In Europe and North America, as of 2014, atrial fibrillation affects about 2% to 3% of the population. Atrial fibrillation and atrial flutter resulted in 112,000 deaths in 2013, up from 29,000 in 1990. However, in most recent cases concerning the SARS-CoV 2 pandemic, cardiac arrhythmias are commonly developed and associated with high morbidity and mortality among patients hospitalized with the COVID-19 infection, due to the infection's ability to cause myocardial injury. Sudden cardiac death is the cause of about half of deaths due to cardiovascular disease and about 15% of all deaths globally. About 80% of sudden cardiac death is the result of ventricular arrhythmias. Arrhythmias may occur at any age but are more common among older people. Arrhythmias may also occur in children; however, the normal range for the heart rate varies with age.

THE BEST AFIB DIETS

The American Heart Association (AHA) recommend that people who experience AFib consume foods low in saturated fats, trans fats, salt, and cholesterol.

A 2017 review found that a plant-based diet high in fruit, vegetables, and whole grains can decrease obesity and hypertension. As these are risk factors for AFib, such dietary measures may help prevent someone from developing the condition.

There is also evidence to suggest that the Mediterranean diet may help reduce the risk of AFib. A 2014 study suggests that olive oil, in particular, is a beneficial part of the diet.

The benefits of the Mediterranean diet for AFib include:

Overall heart health

A study in Circulation Research found that people who follow the Mediterranean diet have better overall heart health compared with those who do not.

Platelet function

Platelets are blood cells that help the body form clots to stop bleeding. A 2015 study found that the Mediterranean diet can positively affect platelet function for people who have AFib.

Lower cholesterol

The Mediterranean diet may lower cholesterol levels. As high cholesterol is a risk factor for AFib, someone who lowers their cholesterol will reduce their chances of developing the condition.

Reduced risk of heart attack and stroke

According to a 2015 study, the Mediterranean diet may reduce the risk of someone with AFib having a heart attack or stroke.

Although these diets may have a positive effect on AFib, if someone wishes to change their food habits, they should discuss their options with a registered dietitian first.

FOODS TO EAT FOR AFIB

The AHA list these foods to eat on the Mediterranean diet:

vegetables

whole grains

olive oil

fruits

legumes

fish

chicken and turkey

nuts and seeds

eggs

dairy

added sugars

highly processed foods

fatty, processed meats
refined carbohydrates

Each meal should contain a good portion of vegetables, a source of protein, a complex carbohydrate, and unsaturated fat. In addition to olive oil, this fat may include avocado oil, flaxseed oil, or hemp seed oil.

If a person needs inspiration for potential meals under the Mediterranean diet, the AHA provide a wide range of recipe ideas.

If a person is vegetarian or vegan, they can follow a more general plant-based diet consisting of vegetables, fruits, whole grains, legumes, and proteins from nonanimal sources.

FOODS TO AVOID FOR AFIB

Foods to avoid may include those that directly trigger symptoms and raise the risk of heart disease and cholesterol. These include:

Caffeine and energy drinks

The AHA recommends that people avoid excessive amounts of caffeine. However, one study found that drinking 1–3 cups of coffee daily may reduce AFib in males. If a person believes that caffeine could be a personal trigger, they may wish to avoid caffeinated foods and drinks, such as coffee and tea.

Alcohol

A 2014 study found that even moderate alcohol intake could be a risk factor for AFib. Therefore, it may be advisable to limit or avoid alcohol.

Red meat

In general, red meats such as beef or lamb tend to have higher amounts of saturated fat than white meat. Saturated fat can raise cholesterol levels, which is a risk factor for AFib. A person who substitutes red meat for plant-based protein may lower their cholesterol levels.

Processed foods

Processed foods, such as ready meals or sausages, tend to have large quantities of salt and preservatives. It may be best to limit the intake of these as they can adversely affect the heart.

Sugary foods and drinks

People should avoid foods and drinks that contain a large amount of sugar, as these can trigger AFib episodes. Sugary foods also increase the risk of heart disease.

Salt

Someone may have more frequent AFib episodes if they consume food with large quantities of salt. Reducing salt intake may be a useful way to help reduce AFib.

If a person follows the Mediterranean diet, they will also need to limit much of the same foods listed above.

There is some evidence that very low carb diets, such as the keto diet, may increase the risk of AFib. However, researchers need to carry out more studies to confirm and understand these findings.

EXERCISE FOR AFIB

In addition to diet, exercise may also help manage AFib risk factors, such as obesity and hypertension.

A 2016 study suggests that people with AFib who exercise regularly have a lower arrhythmia burden than those who do not. This group also had fewer episodes and milder symptoms.

Research suggests that even a small amount of low impact exercise helps reduce the frequency of AFib symptoms.

A person with AFib can consider doing low impact exercises, such as walking, light jogging, or swimming. They should start slowly and build up gradually so they can exercise several times per week.

Some people with AFib may have a pacemaker. A person who has recently had a pacemaker fitted should avoid strenuous exercise for 4–6 weeks. After this time, they can continue most sports and activities, but they must take precautions in contact sports, such as football or boxing. It is also advisable to avoid strenuous sports, including squash.

Anyone with questions about how soon they can take part in sports after having a pacemaker fitted should talk to their healthcare provider.

Other tips for AFib

There are several other ways a person with AFib can adjust their lifestyle to promote heart health.

Quit smoking

People who smoke are 2.1 times more likely to develop AFib. There is also a link between smoking and other diseases, such as coronary artery disease.

Manage sleep conditions

Sleep deprivation, obstructive sleep apnea, and other sleep disorders may increase the risk of AFib coming back after someone has undergone ablation or cardioversion. The management of sleep apnea and stress may help a person improve the quality of their sleep.

Improve relaxation

Stress, anger, and anxiety have a significant effect on AFib. One study reported an 85% drop in AFib symptoms after people reported feeling happy. Regular relaxation and stress reduction through activities like yoga may help someone manage these

emotions.

CHAPTER TWO

AFIB DIET RECIPES

Here are some recipes for AFIB you can try out, the ingredients of each of the recipes are listed alongside the instructions on how to go about the preparations;

Three sisters" wild rice salad

Ingredients

2 ears corn, kernels removed from cob

2 ½ cups diced butternut squash

2 tablespoons olive oil, divided

¼ teaspoon salt, plus more to taste

¾ teaspoon chili powder

1 cup wild rice

1 (15-ounce) can black beans, drained and rinsed

juice of 1 lime

4 ounces queso fresco (can substitute feta), crumbled or diced

Pepper to taste

Instructions

1. Preheat oven to 425°F. Toss the corn kernels and butternut squash with 1 tablespoon of the olive oil, along with the salt and chili powder. Spread the seasoned veggies in a thin layer over a parchment-lined baking sheet and bake for 25-35 minutes, until golden, tossing halfway through.

2. While the veggies are baking, cook wild rice according to package instructions, then drain off any excess water.

3. In a large bowl, combine the cooked wild rice with the roasted corn and squash. Add the black beans, pepper, lime juice, and queso fresco, along with the remaining 1 tablespoon olive oil. Taste and adjust seasoning (salt and pepper) if necessary.

4. Divide into 4 portions, and serve warm or chilled.

Whole wheat pain de mie

Ingredients

1 cup lukewarm milk

1 cup lukewarm water

6 Tbsp butter

2 tsp salt

3 Tbsp sugar

⅓ cup nonfat dry milk

⅓ cup potato flour or heaping ¾ cup potato flakes

5 cups whole white wheat flour

2 ¼ tsp instant yeast

Instructions

Mixing:

1. Combine all of the ingredients, and mix and knead them by hand, mixer, or bread machine to form a smooth, supple dough.

2. Transfer the dough to a lightly greased bowl or dough-rising bucket, cover the bowl or bucket, and allow the dough to rise till puffy though not necessarily doubled in bulk, about 1 ½ hours.

Shaping:

1. Lightly grease a standard (13" x 4" x 4") lidded pain de mie (pullman) pan. Transfer the risen dough to a lightly greased work surface, shape it into a log, and fit it into the pan. Flatten the top as much as possible.

2. Cover the pan with lightly greased plastic wrap, and allow the dough to rise until it's about ½" below the lip of the pan, about 45 minutes.

Baking:

1. Carefully slip the cover onto the pan, and let it rest an additional 15 minutes while you preheat your oven to 350°F. Bake the bread for 25 minutes.

2. Remove the pan from the oven, carefully remove the lid, and return the bread to the oven to bake for an additional 10 to 15 minutes, until it's golden-brown on top and tests done; an instant-read

thermometer inserted into the center will register 190°F.

3. Remove the bread from the oven, and turn it out of the pan onto a rack to cool completely. For a soft, flavorful crust, brush the loaf with melted butter while warm.

Whole wheat sandwich bread

Ingredients

2 ½ tsp active dry yeast or 2 ½ tsp instant yeast

½ cup lukewarm water*

½ cup lukewarm milk

½ cup orange juice

5 Tbsp melted butter

1 ½ tsp salt

3 Tbsp sugar

¼ cup nonfat dry milk

¾ cup instant mashed potato flakes

3 ¾ cups whole wheat flour or white whole wheat flour

*Use 2 Tbsp less water in summer (or in a humid environment), 2 Tbsp more in winter (or in a dry climate).

Instructions

Mixing:

1. Dissolve the yeast in the lukewarm water with a pinch of sugar. Allow it to rest for 15 minutes, till it becomes puffy. If you're using instant yeast, you can skip this step.

2. Combine the yeast/water with the remaining ingredients, and mix and knead by hand, mixer, or bread machine until you've made a cohesive dough. If you're using a stand mixer, knead at low speed for about 7 minutes. Note that 100% whole wheat dough will never become smooth and supple like dough made with all-purpose flour; it'll feel more like clay under your hands, and may appear a bit rough.

Shaping:

1. Place the dough in a lightly greased bowl, cover the bowl, and allow it to rise till it's expanded and looks somewhat puffy, about 60 to 90 minutes. Note that dough kneaded in a bread machine will rise faster and higher than bread kneaded in a mixer, which in turn will rise faster and higher than one

kneaded by hand. So if you're kneading by hand, you may want to let the dough rise longer than 90 minutes.

2. Lightly grease a 9" x 5" loaf pan. Gently shape the dough into a smooth log, and settle it into the pan, smooth side up.

3. Tent the pan with lightly greased plastic wrap, and allow the loaf to rise till it's crowned over the rim of the pan by about ¾", about 75 minutes. Don't let it rise too high; it'll continue to rise as it bakes. Towards the end of the rising time, preheat the oven to 350°F.

Baking:

1. Bake the bread for 10 minutes. Lightly tent it with aluminum foil, and bake for an additional 30 to 35 minutes, or until the center registers 190°F on an

instant-read thermometer. Remove it from the oven, and turn it out of the pan onto a rack.

2. Run a stick of butter over the top of the hot loaf, if desired, for a softer crust. Allow the bread to cool completely before slicing.

Whole grain no-knead bread

Ingredients

200 grams whole wheat flour (about 1 ⅓ cups), plus more for flouring your surface

200 grams all-purpose flour (about 1 ⅓ cups)

340 grams of water (1 ¼ cups + 3 scant tablespoons)

8 grams of salt (about 1 ½ teaspoons table salt, or 2 teaspoons kosher salt)

2 grams instant yeast (about ½ teaspoon)

⅛ teaspoon lemon juice

Instructions

1. Place the whole wheat flour, all-purpose flour, salt, and yeast in a large bowl and stir to combine.

2. Add the water and lemon juice into the flour mixture. With your hand formed in a stiff claw, rake the flour and water together, until it becomes a sticky mass. Roll and press the dough mass around in the bowl to pick up any loose bits of flour. This should take no more than 40 seconds.

3. Cover the bowl with a cutting board or lid and let sit on the counter at room temperature (60-70°F) for 12-18 hours.

4. To shape the loaf, dust one side of a dish towel generously with flour and use it to line a bowl (floured side up). Flour your work surface (such as a countertop) and flour the edges of the dough in the

bowl. This will help the dough slide out of the bowl with minimal sticking. Tilt the bowl over your floured work surface and ease the dough mass out onto your floured countertop.

5. Being gentle with the dough, reach under one side and stretch the dough out slightly, and fold it up and over itself into the center. Repeat this with each side of the dough, so a total of 4 times. Being sure to use as much flour as necessary to prevent sticking, flip the dough over using the sides of your hands (try not to use your fingertips too much). Hold the dough in both hands with the seam side down, and gently tuck the dough together underneath itself, helping to form it into a ball with a relatively smooth top.

6. Place the dough ball seam side down into the towel-lined bowl, and dust lightly with flour. Cover the bowl with a large baking sheet and allow the to rise until roughly doubled in size. This should take about 2 hours. As a test, you can poke the dough with a well-floured finger. If the dent springs back immediately, your dough needs more time to rest. If the dent slowly fills back in you're are ready to bake.

7. Approximately 30 minutes before you think your dough will be ready to bake, place a Dutch oven on the middle rack of your oven, with the lid on. Preheat oven to 500°F. While the oven and Dutch oven are preheating, cut a piece of parchment paper to the size of the loaf. When ready to bake, carefully flip the bowl containing the dough over the prepared piece of parchment paper and gently remove the bowl and the towel from the loaf. Be gentle and

take your time, you want to minimize the loss of gasses from the dough.

8. Carefully remove the (very hot) Dutch oven. Using the corners of the parchment paper, carefully place your loaf inside the vessel. Being sure to use an oven mitt, place the lid back on the Dutch oven and return to the oven, lowering the temperature to 450°F. Bake for 25 minutes. After 25 minutes, remove the lid (be careful of the steam) and bake for 15 to 25 minutes more, or to your desired darkness.

9. Remove the loaf from the Dutch oven and especially because this is a whole grain loaf allow to cool! If you can't wait until it is room temperature, be sure to give it as close to an hour as you can handle before cutting and consuming.

Abc meatball soup

Ingredients

For Meatballs

1 pound extra lean ground turkey breast or 90% lean ground beef

¾ cup oats (quick or old fashioned, uncooked)

⅓ cup barbecue sauce or catsup

For Soup

1 carton (48 ounces) reduced-sodium, fat-free chicken broth (about 6 cups)

¼ cup alphabet-shaped pasta

1 package (10 ounces) frozen mixed vegetables (do not thaw)

Instructions

1. Heat broiler. Lightly spray rack of broiler pan with cooking spray.

2. In a large bowl, combine meatball ingredients; mix lightly but thoroughly. Transfer to a sheet of foil. Pat mixture into 9 x 6-inch rectangle. Cut into 1-½-inch squares; roll each square into a ball to make 24 meatballs. Arrange meatballs on broiler pan.

3. Broil meatballs 6 to 8 inches from heat about 6 minutes or until cooked through, turning once.

4. While meatballs cook, bring chicken broth to a boil in a 4-quart saucepan or Dutch oven over medium-high heat. Add pasta and frozen vegetables; return to boil. Reduce heat; cover and simmer 8 minutes or until vegetables and pasta are tender.

Add meatballs and cook 1 minute. Serve immediately.

Amaranth banana walnut bread

Ingredients

1 cup cooked amaranth

2 cups whole wheat pastry flour

2 tsp. baking powder

½ cup chopped walnuts

1 cup mashed ripe bananas (about 3)

½ cup liquid honey

2 eggs

3 Tbsp melted butter or olive oil

1 tsp. vanilla extract

Instructions

1. Preheat oven to 350°F. Lightly grease a 9-by-5-inch loaf pan.

2. In a bowl, combine flour, baking powder, and walnuts. Mix well. In a separate bowl, beat bananas, honey, eggs, butter, and vanilla until blended. Add amaranth and mix well. Pour mixture over dry ingredients and mix until just combined.

3. Pour mixture into prepared pan. Bake in preheated oven until a tester inserted into the center comes out clean, about 1 hour. Let cool in pan on wire rack for 10 minutes. Remove from pan and let cool completely on rack.

Amaranth cheese grits

Ingredients

1 cup whole grain amaranth

3 cups water

Salt, to taste

1 cup shredded sharp cheddar

3 tablespoons cream cheese

Instructions

1. Combine the water and salt in a large pot and cover with a lid. Bring to a boil. Add whole grain amaranth, cover pot and reduce burner to its lowest setting. Simmer for 20 minutes, or until the water is completely absorbed.

2. Turn off heat, add in the cheddar and cream cheese. Stir well until melted.

Amaranth polenta with wild mushrooms

Ingredients

½ ounce (½ cup loosely packed) dried porcini or other dried mushrooms

1 tablespoon olive oil

¼ cup finely chopped shallots

1 cup amaranth

¼ teaspoon. salt

Freshly ground pepper to taste

1 tsp. chopped fresh thyme, plus more for garnish

Instructions

1. Bring water to a boil in a kettle, and pour 1 ¾ cups boiling water into a large heatproof glass

measuring cup. Stir in the dried mushrooms. Cover and set aside until the mushrooms are soft, about 10 minutes. Chop any large pieces.

2. Meanwhile, heat the olive oil in a heavy 2-quart saucepan. Add the shallots and cook for 1 minute. Stir in the amaranth. Add the soaked mushrooms and the soaking liquid, taking care to leave any grit on the bottom of the cup. Bring to a boil. Reduce the head, cover, and simmer for 15 minutes. Stir in the salt, pepper, and thyme.

3. Continue simmering, covered, until the mixture is porridgy and the amaranth is tender, 10 to 15 minutes more. (Tender amaranth should still be crunchy, but shouldn't taste hard or gritty.) Stir in a bit more boiling water if the mixture becomes too thick before the amaranth is done.

4. Serve in small bowls with a sprinkle of thyme on top.

Amaranth with peppers and cabbage

Ingredients

1 cup uncooked amaranth grains

2 cups water

2 garlic cloves, minced

1 green bell pepper, cored, seeded, and diced

1 poblano pepper (can substitute another bell pepper) cored, seeded, and diced

2 tablespoons extra virgin olive oil

¼ head purple cabbage, chopped into long shreds

salt and pepper to taste

Instructions

1. To cook the amaranth, bring the water and amaranth to a boil, then simmer, partially covered, for 30-35 minutes, until soft, swollen and tender. Remove from the heat and allow to stand for 15 minutes, with the lid still on, to swell more.

2. Meanwhile, in a large shallow pan, gently fry the garlic and diced peppers in the oil until the vegetables are soft.

3. Add the cabbage, season with salt and pepper, and put the lid on to cook for 5 more minutes.

4. Gently stir in the amaranth grains, reheat and serve.

Amaranth-ginger muffins

Ingredients

Liquid Ingredients

2 large eggs, at room temperature

⅔ cup milk

¼ cup canola oil

2 tablespoons molasses (not blackstrap)

1 teaspoon pure vanilla extract

Dry Ingredients

⅔ cup amaranth flour

⅔ cup potato starch

½ cup tapioca flour

1 cup packed dark brown sugar

1 tablespoon baking powder

1 teaspoon xanthan gum

1 teaspooon salt

1 teaspoon ground ginger

1 teaspoon ground cinnamon

½ teaspoon each grated nutmeg and ground allspice

⅛ teaspoon ground cloves

½ cup finely chopped crystallized ginger

¼ cup finely chopped walnuts

Ginger-Sugar Crust

2 tablespoon sugar

½ teaspoon ground ginger

Instructions

1. Place a rack in the middle of the oven. Preheat the oven to 375°F. Generously grease a 12-cup or 6-cup gray nonstick muffin pan or line with paper liners.

2. In a medium bowl, beat the eggs with an electric mixer on medium speed until light yellow and frothy, about 30 seconds. Add the milk, oil, molasses, and vanilla and beat on low speed until well blended.

3. In a small bowl, whisk together the dry ingredients. With the mixer on low speed, gradually beat the dry ingredients into the liquid ingredients until the batter is smooth and slightly thickened. Gently stir in the crystallized ginger and walnuts. Divide the batter evenly in the muffin pan.

4. Make the crust: In a small bowl, whisk together the sugar and ground ginger and sprinkle evenly on the batter.

5. Bake the larger muffins 35 to 40 minutes or the smaller muffins for 20 to 25 minutes or until a toothpick inserted into the center of the muffin comes out clean. Cool the muffins in the pan 10 minutes on a wire rack. Remove the muffins from the pans and cool completely on the wire rack. Serve slightly warm.

Mexican Black Beans and Rice

Ingredients

- 2 tablespoons coconut oil

- 1 teaspoon chili powder

- 1 teaspoon garlic powder

- 1 teaspoon ground cumin

- 1 teaspoon ground coriander

- 2 stalks celery, chopped

- 1 tomato, chopped

- ½ cup frozen corn

- 2 teaspoons chopped fresh oregano

- 2 teaspoons chopped fresh cilantro

- 1 (15 ounce) can black beans, rinsed and drained

- ½ cup mild salsa

- ¼ cup water, or as needed

- 2 cups cooked white rice

- salt to taste

Instructions

- Step 1

Heat coconut oil in a large skillet over medium-low heat. Add chili powder, garlic powder, cumin, and coriander; fry until fragrant, about 30 seconds. Add celery, cook and stir until softened, 3 to 5 minutes.

- Step 2

Add tomato, frozen corn, oregano, and cilantro; stir to coat. Stir in black beans and salsa. Bring to a simmer and cook for 10 to 15 minutes, adding water as needed to keep the mixture saucy.

- Step 3

Remove from the heat and stir in cooked rice until coated. Season with salt.

Instant Pot Baked Beans

Ingredients

- 8 cups water

- 1 pound dry navy beans, rinsed and picked through

- 1 tablespoon olive oil

- 6 ounces salt pork, diced

- 6 ounces bacon, cut into small pieces

- 1 small onion, minced

- 1 ½ cups water, divided

- ¼ cup ketchup

- ⅓ cup molasses

- ¼ cup brown sugar

- 1 tablespoon yellow mustard

Instructions

- Step 1

Combine water and beans in a multi-functional pressure cooker (such as an Instant Pot®). Close and lock the lid. Select high pressure according to manufacturer's instructions; set timer for 15 minutes. Allow 10 to 15 minutes for pressure to build.

- Step 2

Release pressure using the natural-release method for 20 minutes; quick-release remaining pressure according to manufacturer's directions. Unlock and remove the lid. Drain and rinse the beans with cold water and set aside. Rinse and wipe out Instant Pot® insert and place back into the pressure cooker.

- Step 3

Turn on Instant Pot® and select Saute function. Heat olive oil until shimmering, 2 to 3 minutes. Add salt pork, bacon, and onion and briefly cook until fat begins to render, 1 to 2 minutes. Pour in 1/2 cup water and scrape any brown bits off the bottom. Turn Instant Pot® off.

• Step 4

Whisk together ketchup, molasses, brown sugar, mustard, and remaining 1 cup water in a small bowl. Return cooked beans to the pot along with the ketchup mixture. Gently stir to combine. Close and lock the lid. Select high pressure according to manufacturer's instructions; set timer for 35 minutes. Allow 10 to 15 minutes for pressure to build.

• Step 5

Release pressure using the natural-release method for 20 minutes; quick-release any remaining pressure according to manufacturer's directions. Unlock and remove the lid. Beans will thicken upon cooling. Serve immediately or freeze portions for later.

Lentils with Ground Beef and Rice

Ingredients

- 1 cup dry lentils

- 5 cups water

- 1 cube beef bouillon

- ½ cup uncooked white rice

- 3 tablespoons vegetable oil

- 1 medium onion, chopped

- 2 tablespoons chopped red bell pepper

- 2 cloves garlic, minced

- 2 ½ teaspoons ground cumin

- salt and ground black pepper to taste

- 1 pound lean ground beef

- 1 ½ teaspoons ground paprika

Instructions

- Step 1

Place lentils in a bowl and cover with cold water. Soak for at least 4 hours.

- Step 2

Drain lentils and put in a large pot with 5 cups water and bouillon cube; bring to a boil. Reduce heat to a simmer and cook for 15 minutes. Add rice and simmer until rice and lentils are tender, 15 to 20 minutes.

- Step 3

Meanwhile, heat oil in a skillet over medium heat. Add onion, bell pepper, garlic, cumin, salt, and pepper; saute until onion is golden brown and tender, 5 to 7 minutes. Add ground beef; cook and stir until browned and crumbly, 7 to 9 minutes. Add paprika and cook for 1 more minute.

- Step 4

Add meat mixture to lentils and rice. Simmer over low heat for 5 to 10 minutes.

Roasted Sweet Potato, Black Bean, and Chorizo Breakfast Bowls

Ingredients

Sweet Potatoes:

* 2 sweet potatoes, peeled and cut into 1/2-inch cubes

* 1 tablespoon olive oil

* ½ teaspoon ground cumin

* ½ teaspoon salt

Beans:

* 1 (15.5 ounce) can black beans, undrained

* ½ teaspoon ground cumin

* ½ teaspoon salt

* ¼ teaspoon garlic powder

- 1 pound fresh Mexican chorizo sausage, casing removed

- 1 tablespoon butter, or as needed (Optional)

- 4 eggs

- 2 avocados - peeled, pitted, and sliced

Instructions

- Step 1

Preheat the oven to 400 degrees F (200 degrees C). Line a baking sheet with parchment paper.

- Step 2

Combine sweet potatoes, olive oil, cumin, and salt in a medium bowl. Spread evenly on the prepared baking sheet.

- Step 3

Roast in the preheated oven, stirring after 10 minutes, until browned and cooked, 18 to 20 minutes total.

- Step 4

Meanwhile, combine black beans, cumin, salt, and garlic powder in a small saucepan over medium-low heat. Heat until warmed through, 8 to 10 minutes. Keep warm.

- Step 5

Brown chorizo in a large skillet over medium-high heat, breaking up any large clumps, for 5 to 6 minutes. Transfer chorizo to a paper towel-lined plate using a slotted spoon. Reserve about 1 tablespoon grease in the skillet, adding butter as needed to make up the difference.

- Step 6

Crack eggs into the skillet and cook until whites are set and yolks reach the desired doneness, 3 to 5 minutes.

- Step 7

Divide sweet potatoes, drained black beans, chorizo, and avocados between 4 bowls. Top each bowl with an egg.

Indian Kale with Chickpeas

Ingredients

- 2 tablespoons olive oil, or as needed

- 1 onion, finely chopped

- 1 red chile pepper, seeded and sliced

- 1 (14 ounce) can chickpeas, drained

- 1 tablespoon ground cumin

- 1 teaspoon ground coriander

- ½ teaspoon ground turmeric

- 1 pinch ground cinnamon

- 1 pinch sea salt

- 1 lemon, zested and juiced

- 1 cup roughly chopped kale, or more to taste

Instructions

- Step 1

Heat oil in a large frying pan or wok over medium-high heat. Add onion and chile pepper; saute until onion is tender, 5 to 7 minutes. Add chickpeas, cumin, coriander, turmeric, cinnamon, and salt; saute for 5 minutes. Pour in a splash of water, followed by lemon zest and juice. Season further to taste if desired.

- Step 2

Fold kale into the mixture until just wilted, 3 to 5 minutes. Remove from heat and serve.

Frijoles de Olla

Ingredients

- 10 cups water

- 2 tablespoons lard

- 2 cups dry pinto beans, rinsed

- 2 teaspoons salt

Instructions

- Step 1

Measure water and lard into a large pot. Bring to a boil and add beans. Cook over medium heat for 2 to 2 1/2 hours. Season with salt and continue cooking until tender, about 30 more minutes.

Creamy salmon, leek & potato traybake

Ingredients

• 250g baby potatoes , thickly sliced

• 2 tbsp olive oil

• 1 leek , halved, washed and sliced

• 1 garlic clove , crushed

• 70ml double cream

• 1 tbsp capers , plus extra to serve

• 1 tbsp chives , plus extra to serve

• 2 skinless salmon fillets

• mixed rocket salad , to serve (optional)

Instructions

• STEP 1

Heat the oven to 200C/180C fan/gas 6. Bring a medium pan of water to the boil. Add the potatoes and cook for 8 mins. Drain and leave to steam-dry in a colander for a few minutes. Toss the potatoes with ½ of the oil and plenty of seasoning in a baking tray. Put in the oven for 20 mins, tossing halfway through the cooking time.

• STEP 2

Meanwhile, heat the remaining oil in a frying pan over a medium heat. Add the leek and fry for 5 mins, or until beginning to soften. Stir through the garlic for 1 min, then add the cream, capers and 75ml hot water, then bring to the boil. Stir through the chives.

• STEP 3

Heat the grill to high. Pour the creamy leek mixture over the potatoes, then sit the salmon fillets on top. Grill for 7-8 mins, or until just cooked through. Serve topped with extra chives and capers and a salad on the side, if you like.

Curried cod

Ingredients

• 1 tbsp oil

• 1 onion, chopped

• 2 tbsp medium curry powder

• thumb-sized piece ginger, peeled and finely grated

- 3 garlic cloves, crushed

- 2 x 400g cans chopped tomatoes

- 400g can chickpeas

- 4 cod fillets (about 125-150g each)

- zest 1 lemon, then cut into wedges

- handful coriander, roughly chopped

Instructions

- STEP 1

Heat the oil in a large, lidded frying pan. Cook the onion over a high heat for a few mins, then stir in the curry powder, ginger and garlic. Cook for another 1-2 mins until fragrant, then stir in the tomatoes, chickpeas and some seasoning.

- STEP 2

Cook for 8-10 mins until thickened slightly, then top with the cod. Cover and cook for another 5-10 mins until the fish is cooked through. Scatter over the lemon zest and coriander, then serve with the lemon wedges to squeeze over.

Easy fish pie recipe

Ingredients

• 1kg Maris Piper potatoes, peeled and halved

• 400ml milk, plus a splash

• 25g butter, plus a knob

• 25g plain flour

• 4 spring onions, finely sliced

• 1 x pack fish pie mix (cod, salmon, smoked haddock etc, weight around 320g-400g depending on pack size)

• 1 tsp Dijon or English mustard

• ½ a 25g pack or a small bunch chives, finely snipped

• handful frozen sweetcorn

• handful frozen petits pois

• handful grated cheddar

Instructions

• STEP 1

Heat the oven to 200C/fan 180C/gas mark 6.

• STEP 2

Put 1kg potatoes, peeled and halved, in a saucepan and pour over enough water to cover them. Bring to the boil and then simmer until tender.

• STEP 3

When cooked, drain thoroughly and mash with a splash of milk and a knob of butter. Season with ground black pepper.

• STEP 4

Put 25g butter, 25g plain flour and 4 finely sliced spring onions in another pan and heat gently until the butter has melted, stirring regularly. Cook for 1-2 mins.

• STEP 5

Gradually whisk in 400ml milk using a balloon whisk if you have one. Bring to the boil, stirring to avoid any lumps and sticking at the bottom of the pan. Cook for 3-4 mins until thickened.

• STEP 6

Take off the heat and stir in 320g-400g mixed fish, 1 tsp Dijon or English mustard, a small bunch of finely snipped chives, handful of sweetcorn and handful of petits pois. Spoon into an ovenproof dish or 6-8 ramekins.

• STEP 7

Spoon the potato on top and sprinkle with a handful of grated cheddar cheese.

• STEP 8

Pop in the oven for 20-25 mins or until golden and bubbling at the edges. Alternatively, cover and freeze the pie or mini pies for another time.

Chorizo, new potato & haddock one-pot

Ingredients

• 1 tbsp extra-virgin olive oil , plus extra to serve

• 50g chorizo , peeled and thinly sliced

• 450g salad or new potatoes , sliced (I used Charlotte)

• 4 tbsp dry sherry , or more if you need it (or use white wine)

• 2 skinless thick fillets white fish (I used sustainably caught haddock)

• good handful cherry tomatoes , halved

• 20g bunch parsley , chopped

• crusty bread , to serve

Instructions

• STEP 1

Heat a large lidded frying pan, then add the oil. Tip in the chorizo, fry for 2 mins until it starts to release its oils, then tip in the potatoes and some seasoning. Splash over 3 tbsp sherry, cover the pan tightly, then leave to cook for 10-15 mins until the potatoes are just tender. Move them around the pan a bit halfway through.

• STEP 2

Season the fish well. Give the potatoes another stir, add the cherry tomatoes and most of the chopped parsley to the pan, then lay the fish on top. Splash over 1 tbsp sherry, put the lid on again, then leave to cook for 5 mins, or until the fish has turned white and is flaky when prodded in the middle. Scatter the whole dish with a little more parsley and drizzle with more extra virgin oil. Serve straight away with crusty bread.

Superhealthy salmon burgers

Ingredients

• 4 boneless, skinless salmon fillets, about 550g/1lb 4oz in total, cut into chunks

• 2 tbsp Thai red curry paste

• thumb-size piece fresh root ginger, grated

• 1 tsp soy sauce

• 1 bunch coriander, half chopped, half leaves picked

• 1 tsp vegetable oil

• lemon wedges, to serve

For the salad

• 2 carrots

• half large or 1 small cucumber

• 2 tbsp white wine vinegar

• 1 tsp golden caster sugar

Instructions

• STEP 1

Tip the salmon into a food processor with the paste, ginger, soy and chopped coriander. Pulse until roughly minced. Tip out the mix and shape into 4 burgers. Heat the oil in a non-stick frying pan, then fry the burgers for 4-5 mins on each side, turning until crisp and cooked through.

• STEP 2

Meanwhile, use a swivel peeler to peel strips of carrot and cucumber into a bowl. Toss with the vinegar and sugar until the sugar has dissolved, then toss through the coriander leaves. Divide the salad between 4 plates. Serve with the burgers and rice.

Smoky hake, beans & greens

Ingredients

• mild olive oil

• ½ x 200g pack raw cooking chorizo (we used Unearthed Alfresco Smoked)

• 1 onion, finely chopped

• 260g bag spinach

• 2 x 140g skinless hake fillets

• ½ tsp sweet smoked paprika

• 1 red chilli, deseeded and shredded

• 400g can cannellini beans, drained

• juice ½ lemon

• 1 tbsp extra virgin olive oil

To serve

• Quick garlic mayonnaise (optional) - see recipe in tip

Instructions

• STEP 1

Boil a full kettle of water and heat the grill to high. Heat 1 tsp oil in a large frying pan. Squeeze the meat from the chorizo directly into the pan. Add the onion and fry for 5 mins, crushing the meat with a spatula until broken up, golden and surrounded by its juices. The onion will also be soft and golden.

• STEP 2

Meanwhile, put the spinach in a colander, slowly pour over the boiled water to wilt it, then run under the cold tap. Squeeze out the excess water using your hands, then set aside. Line a baking tray with foil, rub with a little oil and place the fish on top. Season, sprinkle over the smoked paprika and drizzle with a little more oil.

• STEP 3

Tip the chilli into the pan with the sausages, fry for 1 min more, then add the beans, spinach, lemon juice and extra virgin olive oil. Let it warm through gently, then season to taste.

• STEP 4

Grill the fish for 5 mins or until flaky but not dry – you won't need to turn it. Spoon the bean mixture onto plates, then carefully top with the fish and any juices from the tray. Serve with a dollop of Quick

garlic mayonnaise (see recipe, right), if you like.

Smoky hake, beans & greens

Ingredients

• mild olive oil

• ½ x 200g pack raw cooking chorizo (we used

Unearthed Alfresco Smoked)

• 1 onion, finely chopped

• 260g bag spinach

• 2 x 140g skinless hake fillets

• ½ tsp sweet smoked paprika

• 1 red chilli, deseeded and shredded

• 400g can cannellini beans, drained

• juice ½ lemon

• 1 tbsp extra virgin olive oil

To serve

• Quick garlic mayonnaise (optional) - see recipe in
tip

Instructions

• STEP 1

Boil a full kettle of water and heat the grill to high.
Heat 1 tsp oil in a large frying pan. Squeeze the
meat from the chorizo directly into the pan. Add the
onion and fry for 5 mins, crushing the meat with a
spatula until broken up, golden and surrounded by
its juices. The onion will also be soft and golden.

• STEP 2

Meanwhile, put the spinach in a colander, slowly
pour over the boiled water to wilt it, then run under

the cold tap. Squeeze out the excess water using your hands, then set aside. Line a baking tray with foil, rub with a little oil and place the fish on top. Season, sprinkle over the smoked paprika and drizzle with a little more oil.

• STEP 3

Tip the chilli into the pan with the sausages, fry for 1 min more, then add the beans, spinach, lemon juice and extra virgin olive oil. Let it warm through gently, then season to taste.

• STEP 4

Grill the fish for 5 mins or until flaky but not dry – you won't need to turn it. Spoon the bean mixture onto plates, then carefully top with the fish and any juices from the tray. Serve with a dollop of Quick garlic mayonnaise (see recipe, right), if you like.

Simple seafood chowder

Ingredients

• 1 tbsp vegetable oil

• 1 large onion, chopped

• 100g streaky bacon, chopped

• 1 tbsp plain flour

• 600ml fish stock, made from 1 fish stock cube

• 225g new potato, halved

• pinch mace

• pinch cayenne pepper

• 300ml milk

• 320g pack fish pie mix (salmon, haddock and smoked haddock)

• 4 tbsp single cream

* 250g pack cooked mixed shellfish

* small bunch parsley, chopped

* crusty bread, to serve

Instructions

* STEP 1

Heat the oil in a large saucepan over a medium heat, then add the onion and bacon. Cook for 8-10 mins until the onion is soft and the bacon is cooked. Stir in the flour, then cook for a further 2 mins.

* STEP 2

Pour in the fish stock and bring it up to a gentle simmer. Add the potatoes, cover, then simmer for 10-12 mins until the potatoes are cooked through.

* STEP 3

Add the mace, cayenne pepper and some seasoning, then stir in the milk.

• STEP 4

Tip the fish pie mix into the pan, gently simmer for 4 mins. Add the cream and shellfish, then simmer for 1 min more. Check the seasoning. Sprinkle with the parsley and serve with some crusty bread.

Ultimate fish cakes

Ingredients

For the tartare-style sauce

• 125ml mayonnaise

• 1 rounded tbsp capers, roughly chopped (rinsed and drained if salted)

• 1 rounded tsp creamed horseradish

• 1 rounded tsp Dijon mustard

• 1 small shallot, very finely chopped

• 1 tsp flatleaf parsley, finely chopped

For the fish cakes

• 450g skinned Icelandic cod or haddock fillet, from

a sustainable source

• 2 bay leaves

• 150ml milk

• 350g Maris Piper potatoes

• ½ tsp finely grated lemon zest

• 1 tbsp flatleaf parsley, chopped

• 1 tbsp snipped chives

• 1 egg

* flour, for shaping

* 85g fresh white breadcrumbs, preferably a day or two old

* 3-4 tbsp vegetable or sunflower oil, for shallow frying

* lemon wedges and watercress, to serve

Instructions

* STEP 1

Mix together 125ml mayonnaise, 1 rounded tbsp roughly chopped capers, 1 rounded tsp creamed horseradish, 1 rounded tsp Dijon mustard, 1 small very finley chopped shallot and 1 tsp finely chopped flatleaf parsley. Set aside.

• STEP 2

Lay 450g skinned Icelandic cod or haddock fillet and 2 bay leaves in a frying pan. Pour over 150ml milk and 150ml water.

• STEP 3

Cover, bring to a boil, then lower the heat and simmer for 4 mins. Take off the heat and let stand, covered, for 10 mins to gently finish cooking the fish.

• STEP 4

Meanwhile, peel and chop 350g Maris Piper potatoes into even-sized chunks. Put them in a saucepan and just cover with boiling water. Add a pinch of salt, bring back to the boil and simmer for 10 mins or until tender, but not broken up.

- STEP 5

Lift the fish out of the milk with a slotted spoon and put on a plate to cool. Drain the potatoes in a colander and leave for a min or two.

- STEP 6

Tip the potatoes back into the hot pan on the lowest heat you can and let them dry out for 1 min, mashing them with a fork and stirring so they don't stick. You should have a light, dry fluffy mash.

- STEP 7

Take off the heat and beat in 1 rounded tbsp of the sauce, then ½ tsp lemon zest, 1 tbsp chopped flatleaf parsley and 1 tbsp snipped chives.

- STEP 8

Season well with salt and pepper. The potato should have a good flavour, so taste and adjust to suit.

• STEP 9

Drain off liquid from the fish, grind some pepper over it, then flake it into big chunks into the pan of potatoes.

• STEP 10

Using your hands, gently lift the fish and potatoes together so they just mix. You'll only need a couple of turns, or the fish will break up too much. Put to one side and cool.

• STEP 11

Beat 1 egg on a large plate and lightly flour a board. Spread 85g fresh white breadcrumbs on a baking sheet. Divide the fish cake mixture into four.

• STEP 12

On the floured board, and with floured hands, carefully shape into four cakes, about 2.5cm thick. One by one, sit each cake in the egg, and brush over the top and sides so it is completely coated.

• STEP 13

Sit the cakes on the crumbs, patting the crumbs on the sides and tops so they are lightly covered. Transfer to a plate, cover and chill for 30 mins (or up to a day ahead).

• STEP 14

Heat 3-4 tbsp vegetable or sunflower oil in a large frying pan. To test when ready, drop a piece of the dry breadcrumbs in - if it sizzles and quickly turns golden brown, it is ready to use.

• STEP 15

Fry the fish cakes over a medium heat for about 5 mins on each side or until crisp and golden. Serve with the rest of the sauce (squeeze in a little lemon to taste), lemon wedges for squeezing over and watercress.

Easiest ever paella

Ingredients

• 1 tbsp olive oil

• 1 leek or onion, sliced

• 110g pack chorizo sausage, chopped

• 1 tsp turmeric

• 300g long grain rice

• 1l hot fish or chicken stock

• 200g frozen pea

• 400g frozen seafood mix, defrosted

Instructions

• STEP 1

Heat the oil in a deep frying pan, then soften the leek for 5 mins without browning. Add the chorizo and fry until it releases its oils. Stir in the turmeric and rice until coated by the oils, then pour in the stock. Bring to the boil, then simmer for 15 mins, stirring occasionally.

• STEP 2

Tip in the peas and cook for 5 mins, then stir in the seafood to heat through for a final 1-2 mins cooking or until rice is cooked. Check for seasoning and serve immediately with lemon wedges.

Slow cooker chicken pot pie

Ingredients

• 1 to 1 1/2 pounds boneless skinless chicken (thighs or breast meat)

• 4 cups cubed potatoes

• 2 cups peeled and diced carrots

• 2 cups green beans (raw, canned, or frozen all work)

• 3 cups chicken stock

• 1 onion diced, about 1 cup

• 1 teaspoon salt

• 1 teaspoon black pepper

- 1/2 teaspoon garlic powder

- 1/2 teaspoon rubbed sage

- 1 cup cream

- prepared biscuits (I recommend this easy biscuit recipe)

Instructions

1. In the bowl of your slow cooked add the chicken, potatoes, onions, carrots, green beans, stock, onion, and spices.

2. Add the lid and allow to cook until the vegetables are tender and the meat is cooked through, 4-6 hours on high or 6-8 hours on low.

3. Towards the end of your cooking time make your biscuits.

4. When the meat is cooked remove it from the slow cooker and shred it well. Return the meat to the slow cooker and stir to combine.

5. Add the cream and stir well.

6. Add salt and pepper to taste and serve with fresh biscuits on top.

Chicken piccata

Ingredients

• 2 lemons

• ½ cup all-purpose flour

• 4 boneless, skinless chicken breasts

• Salt and pepper

• ¼ cup vegetable oil

• 1 shallot, minced

• 1 garlic clove, minced

• 1 cup chicken broth

• 2 tablespoons capers, rinsed

• 3 tablespoons unsalted butter, cut into pieces and chilled

• 2 tablespoons fresh parsley, minced

Instructions

1. Adjust oven rack to middle position and heat oven to 200°F. Halve 1 lemon, trim ends, and slice lemon into thin half-moons. With the remaining lemon, squeeze ¼ cup juice.

2. Cut chicken horizontally into 2 thin cutlets, then cover with plastic wrap and pound to ½-inch thickness.

3. Pat cutlets dry with paper towels. Season with salt and pepper.

4. Dredge chicken in flour, shaking off any excess.

5. Heat 2 tablespoons oil in large skillet over medium-high heat. Heat oil until just smoking.

6. Brown half of the chicken cutlets until lightly golden on both sides (about 4 minutes).

7. Transfer to plate and keep warm in the oven. Repeat with remaining oil and cutlets.

8. Add shallot and garlic to the oil left in the skillet and cook over medium heat until shallot is softened (about 2 minutes).

9. Stir in broth and lemon slices. Scrape up any browned bits and simmer until reduced and slightly syrupy (about 8 minutes).

10. Stir in lemon juice and capers. Turn the heat to low and whisk in putter, 1 piece at a time.

11. Turn off heat, stir in parsley, and season with salt and pepper.

12. Spoon sauce over chicken and serve.

Sheet pan chicken fajitas

Ingredients

- 2 teaspoons chili powder

- 1 teaspoon garlic powder

- 1 teaspoon smoked paprika

- 1 teaspoon cumin

- 1 teaspoon salt

- ½ teaspoon ground black pepper

• 1 ½ pounds boneless skinless chicken, cut into ½-inch slices

• 1 tablespoon olive oil

• 3 large bell peppers, cut into strips (any colors you prefer)

• 1 medium white onion, cut into thin strips

• Juice of 1 lime

• 2 tablespoons chopped cilantro, optional

• 12 small corn or flour tortillas for serving

• Lime wedges, sour cream, grated cheese, guacamole, optional for serving

Instructions

1. Preheat the oven to 400 degrees F., and spray a large rimmed baking sheet with cooking spray (the baking sheet should be roughly 17×12 inches).

2. In a small bowl, add the chili powder, garlic powder, smoked paprika, cumin, salt, and pepper. Stir well to combine and set aside.

3. Add the chicken to the sheet pan and drizzle with the olive oil.

4. Sprinkle the seasoning mixture over the chicken, and toss well to combine.

5. Add the bell peppers and onion to the sheet pan, and toss gently to combine.

6. Bake until the chicken is cooked through, about 20 minutes. Check a few of the largest pieces to make sure they register 165 degrees F. on an instant-read thermometer.

7. When the chicken is cooked, remove from the oven.

8. Toss lightly to combine again.

9. Drizzle the pan with the juice of 1 lime and sprinkle with chopped cilantro if using.

10. Serve in warmed tortillas with additional toppings of your choice.

Easy Stir Fry Vegetables

Ingredients

For the vegetables

- 1 1/2 pounds (2 large heads) broccoli

- 1 head broccolini (or 1 additional head of broccoli)

- 1 medium red onion

- 1 orange bell pepper

- 2 portobello mushroom caps

For the stir fry sauce

- 3 garlic cloves

- 2 teaspoons ginger, grated (about a 2-inch nub)

- 2 tablespoons mirin

- 2 tablespoons rice vinegar

- 2 tablespoons soy sauce

- 1 teaspoon Sriracha hot sauce

- 2 tablespoons sesame oil (regular, not toasted)

- Kosher salt

For serving

• Garnish: Sliced green onion, sesame seeds (optional)

• Protein: Add ¾ cup cashews with the broccoli*, 1 cup shelled edamame after 2 minutes, or serve with Marinaded Tofu or Sauteed Shrimp (with sesame oil and lime)

• Rice: Rice or Instant Pot Rice, to serve

Instructions

1. Start the rice and decide which protein you'll be adding.

2. Chop the broccoli and broccolini into large florets (about 6 cups florets total). Chop the red onion into bite sized squares. Dice the pepper into bite sized squares. Remove the stems from the portobellos (if necessary), slice them into strips,

then cut the larger pieces in half. Place all of the vegetables in a large bowl.

3. Mince the garlic. Peel the ginger and grate it. Place them together in a small bowl.

4. Stir together the mirin, rice vinegar, soy sauce, and Sriracha in a small bowl.

5. In a large skillet or wok over high heat, and heat the oil. Add the broccoli, broccolini (if using), red onion, bell pepper, and mushrooms and cook 6 to 7 minutes until just starting to brown on edges, stirring occasionally.

6. Add the garlic and ginger cook for 1 minute more, until broccoli is crisp tender but still bright green. Turn off the heat and add the sauce, stirring until combined. Taste and add additional pinches salt as necessary. Garnish with sesame seeds and green

onion (optional). Serve with rice and desired protein (see above).

Epic Roasted Broccoli

Ingredients

• 1 1/2 pounds fresh broccoli, stem on (about 3 large heads or 6 heaping cups florets)

• 3 tablespoons olive oil, divided

• ½ teaspoon kosher salt

• Fresh ground pepper

• 1 medium garlic clove

• 2 tablespoons fresh lemon juice

Instructions

1. Preheat the oven to 450 degrees Fahrenheit. Line a baking sheet with parchment paper.

2. Chop the broccoli into medium-sized florets, leaving a good amount of the stem for a nice shape (see the photo). Mix the broccoli florets with 2 tablespoons olive oil and the kosher salt. Roast for 20 to 25 minutes, until tender and slightly browned (no need to stir!).

3. When the broccoli is done, remove the pan from the oven. Grate the garlic onto the pan, and add the remaining 1 tablespoon olive oil and the lemon juice. Use a spoon to gently toss it all together (separating any grated garlic that clumps together). Serve immediately.

Perfect Sauteed Carrots

Ingredients

• 8 medium carrots (1 pound)

• 2 tablespoons olive oil

• ¼ teaspoon plus 1 pinch kosher salt

• 1 tablespoon chopped fresh thyme (or other fresh herbs — we used a combination of thyme and chives)

Instructions

1. Peel the carrots and slice them diagonally into rounds (on the bias).

2. Heat the olive oil in a large skillet over medium high heat. Add the carrots and cover. Cook for 4 minutes without stirring.

3. Remove the lid, stir, and add the ¼ teaspoon kosher salt. Continue to saute uncovered 3 to 4 minutes until browned, stirring occasionally. Remove from the heat and stir in the fresh herbs and a few more pinches kosher salt to taste. Serve immediately.

Celery Salad With Apples

Ingredients

- 8 celery ribs plus ½ cup celery leaves

- 1 red apple

- 1 tablespoon white wine vinegar

- ½ tablespoon Dijon mustard

- 1 teaspoon maple syrup or sugar

- ½ teaspoon kosher salt

- 3 tablespoons olive oil

• ¼ cup shaved Parmesan cheese

Instructions

1. Thinly slice the celery ribs. Measure out the celery leaves. Thinly slice the red apple.

2. In a medium bowl, whisk together the white wine vinegar, Dijon mustard, maple syrup or sugar, and kosher salt. Gradually whisk in the olive oil one tablespoon at a time.

3. In another bowl, toss together the celery and celery leaves with the apple, dressing, and Parmesan cheese shavings. Serve immediately or refrigerate until serving. This tastes best the day of making, but you can refrigerate leftovers for a few days (refresh them with a little vinegar or salt if necessary).

CHAPTER THREE

SUMMARY

AFib causes an irregular heartbeat. Several risk factors, such as obesity, high blood pressure, and diabetes, make it more likely that a person will develop AFib.

Diet can help reduce the risk factors that cause AFib and, in some cases, reduce its symptoms. The Mediterranean diet or a plant-based diet with plenty of fruits, vegetables, and unsaturated fats may benefit overall heart health, lower cholesterol, and reduce the risk of a heart attack.

Other changes that may improve AFib include doing moderate exercise several times per week, getting high quality sleep, stopping smoking, and prioritizing time to relax and reduce stress.